DEALING WITH STRESS

ANTHONY EKANEM

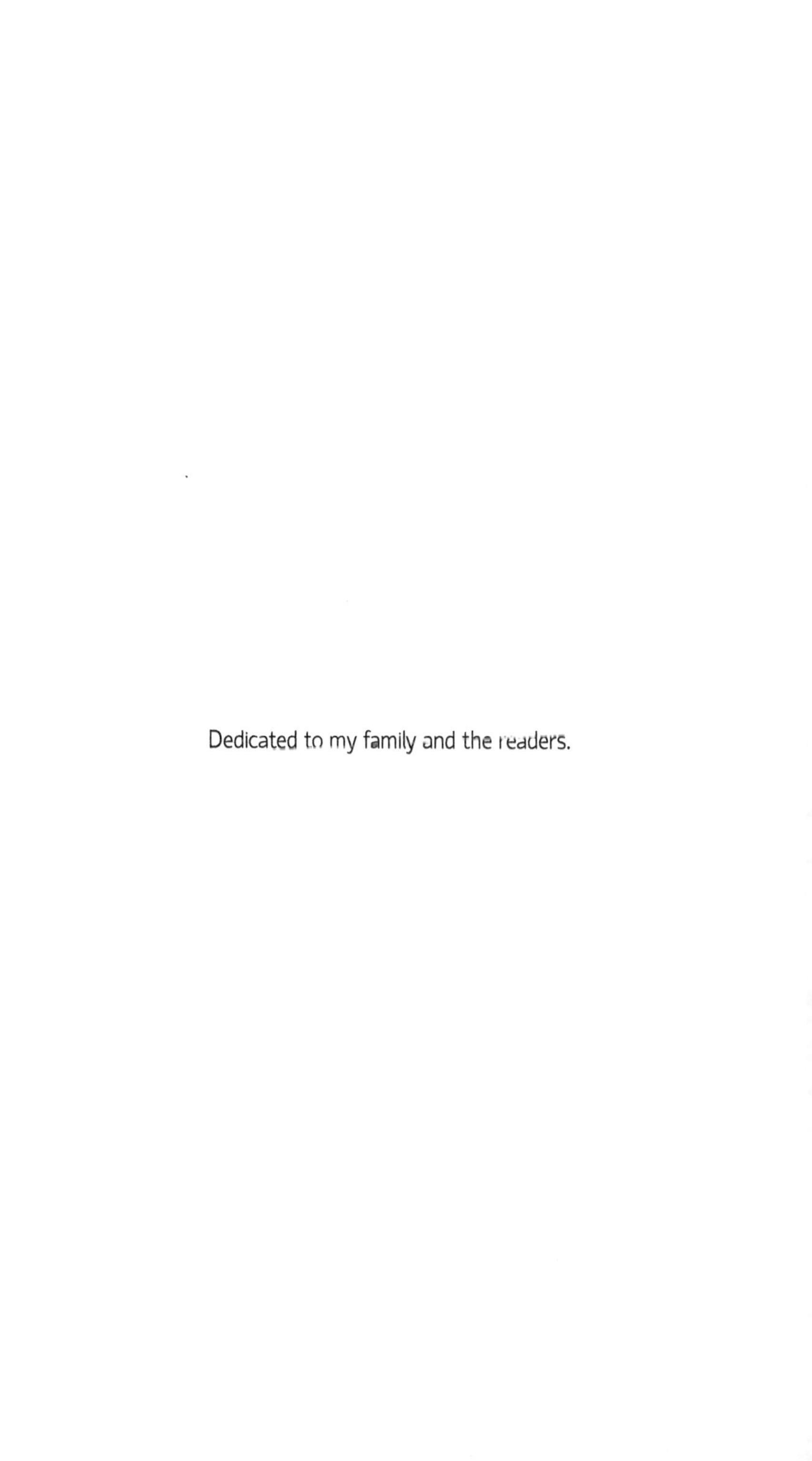

Dedicated to my family and the readers.

Contents

Preface

There is no exact measure or definition of stress, but it is generally defined as the physical and normal response of the body to things that makes them feel worried and bothered. Stress affects individuals differently; the same way individuals view stress in different ways. Indeed, stress is already part of life, and it can strike at any point in one's life.

Though stress can happen inevitably, many individuals still desire not to allow stress to rule their entire system. It is for this reason that individuals make stress resolutions to finally get over this unwanted feeling. Before individuals make resolutions, they tend to look back on the previous years and determine if things went out the way they should be. Individuals start to make resolutions to resolve weight problems, eliminate stress and more.

Stress resolutions are made by individuals who no longer want to be tied with this bothering feeling. When one makes a resolution, they begin to envision a new year where things will fall into place. Embracing these resolutions is synonymous with making commitments and doing the very best to succeed. If you are looking forward to a different and stress-free life, stress resolutions can serve as your guide and inspiration.

These resolutions also help you in living a happier and healthier life. It is true that making life changes requires effort and dedication and starting this journey to change by making stress resolutions are a brilliant step to take. No one ever desires to live a life full of chaos and stress therefore making stress resolutions becomes a top priority of many individuals from different walks of life.

Individuals aspiring for a big change in their life must be familiar with the stress resolutions basics. The first step to take is planning and taking down notes on paper.

Create resolutions and write these down and determine the best ways to fulfil all your goals. You are also tasked to make periodic assessments to determine where your resolutions are taking you. If you are living a stressful life, the first resolution should be identifying where majorities of stress are coming from, and the rest will follow.

CHAPTER ONE

Understand What Stresses You

Stress may affect individuals in many ways, and these may affect their personal and professional life. Regardless of the things or event that stresses you, it is more important to have the willingness and determination to overcome them. It is essential to understand what stresses you because it is only then that you will be able to move forward and avoid these stressful things or events completely. The following might be one of the causes of stress affecting many individuals these days:

Work

Heavy workloads are just one of the many things that cause individuals' stress. Work stress and pressures are common these days and experienced by many employees and working professionals. Doing tons of work for a longer period, meeting deadlines and many other work-related issues can trigger stress.

Work can cause stress if you are already unhappy with it or you are given heavy workloads and too much responsibility. Other factors that can cause stress in work are poor management, unclear work expectations, lack of involvement in making decisions, and more. Working under pressure and complicated conditions and experiencing discrimination also trigger stress.

Money Matters

Financial issues are what stress many people, and these are among the many factors that can cause headaches if not properly addressed. In some instances, individuals are left in stressful and hopeless situations because they are left with no means during the time that they are desperately in need of money. In other cases, a limited budget is also what causes stress. There might be a source of income, but the amount of money earned may not be enough to cover the growing needs.

Family Problems

Problems and conflicts within the family also cause stress. Living under one roof where harmony and strong family ties no longer prevail can be stressful and devastating. Having arguments with your parents and siblings does not just stress you out but also affects you emotionally. Family problems can also interfere with your normal function at home or in the workplace.

Complicated Relationship

One of the most common things that trigger stress is complicated relationships. Unfaithful partners and many other relationship issues tend to break couples apart and this leads to never-ending stress.

There are more other real-life scenarios that cause stress and hopelessness to individuals. The things that generally stop individuals from living a happy and satisfying life that they are dreaming of are the following:

- Loved one's death
- Heavy financial obligations
- Divorce

- Marriage
- Lack of job
- Relocation
- Injury or chronic illness
- Emotional problems such as anger, grief, low self-confidence, and guilt.

CHAPTER TWO

Understand Who Stresses You

Some individuals cause you stress and can give you a terrible headache. Living with people who are also stressed entails a higher possibility of being stressed too. It is essential to know destructive people who stress you and as much as possible let go of them. The following are the individuals who cause you stress:

Viral People

They are termed as such because they seem to appear like bad flu. These are people who always cause discord in your life. Viral people are those who cannot manage to be happy unless there are things and events to hate. These types of individuals can be stressful. After visiting or hanging out with them, you certainly feel drained as if you are having a terrible cold.

Attention Seekers

Individuals who are always messing around and destructing their routines can also cause stress. These are the types of people who wanted the world to revolve around them as much as possible. What can be stressing, and bothering is when they tend to demand all your time and attention and get mad when you fail to give them what they want.

Victim Players

Victim players are those who blamed themselves when something wrong happens. Some individuals might view life's ups and downs as normal events, but victim players see dark phases of their life as the end of the world. Hanging out with these types of people can cause stress and can bring life with negative vibes. As much as possible, get rid of these individuals for they will just interfere with your normal and happy life.

Mental Abusers and Bullies

Bullies are not just dominant during your childhood years because even during adulthood you can still encounter bullies and mental abusers. These types of people are anywhere to be found. They may be present in the neighbourhood, at school or in the workplace. Mingling with these individuals can cause you stress and other worst effects. Aside from being stressed out, bullies and mental abusers are the reasons while others are living in fear.

Having to deal with them can upset a person and this is what seems to be stressful on their part. Mental abusers can be your ex-wife or husband, significant other or worst, they can be your parents. Studies revealed that increased numbers of younger children are living stressful and complicated lives because they are suffering from mental and physical abuse from their parents.

Floaters

The reason why floaters fall under the "Who Stresses You" category is that they would just surprisingly come out when they need help. They may appear right in front of you if they need food or shelter. Of course, it is great to help others, however, it can start to be stressing and annoying if these attitudes and behaviour become a way of life for these types of individuals. When floaters are no longer welcome, they start to find another who can help them.

In general, those who stresses you are those who got negative behaviour and influences. These are people who exclude or ignore you, give you unachievable tasks and set you up just to see you fail. Stressing people are also those who spread malicious gossip and rumours about you, make offending and insulting remarks, underestimate your talents and potentials and undermine your integrity.

Those who stress you are those who deliberately withhold information that you deserve or need to know, make you look so stupid in public and fail to give you due credit for your essential contribution. Let go of these people or else you will notice yourself eventually drowning in pessimistic life with them. Getting rid of them completely entails a stress-free life, the type of life that you deserve.

CHAPTER THREE

Get the Acceptance Mindset

There are inevitable instances that individuals are frustrated and stressed out. Stress is a natural response and having such a feeling is normal. Experts revealed that stress is of two kinds, good stress, and bad stress.

The former is said to be the type that is motivating and beneficial while the latter is causing health problems and anxiety. Little doses of stress are good for it motivates individuals to be better, energize them and inspire them to be more productive and efficient. However, there starts to be a problem when stress is recurring and is staying in one's life for a longer period.

The Right Mindset

The key to overcoming the worst scenarios caused by stress is to get the acceptance mindset. When you are up to something, you must accept that there are things that are not meant for you.

The more you insist, the more things get complicated. What matters is you do your best and achieve results. Simple as they may be, they are considered the fruits of your hard work and perseverance. Do not be stressed out when you failed to achieve the peak for you are always given all the chances to grow and be better as a person.

The acceptance mindset can make you feel at ease and relieved. You do not have to occupy yourself asking why things did not happen the way you want them to be because this can be stressful on your part. You also must accept that you are not an exemption because somewhere along the way, you might experience stress the way others are experiencing this. The best approach for this is to determine the major sources of your stress and deal with them the right way.

You must accept that stress is already part of life and chances are you might be one of the victims. It is all up to you if you wanted to stay in the trap or get out of it completely. Cultivating the proper mindset is an essential part of your stress management. Achieving your goals and desire for a stress-free and happy life takes plenty of effort, determination, and an ideal mindset. However, some individuals will be sabotaging your effort by bringing distorted thoughts, so you must be very careful.

To eliminate stress from your system, stop resisting and believe in the power of an acceptance mindset. You might observe others stuck in the most stressful scenarios of their life without even thinking that these may also happen to you. But in case you have been victimized by stress, you must accept this and convince yourself that unpredictable things happen, and these are all part of life's beauty and complexities.

CHAPTER FOUR

Practice Breathing Exercises

Stressed individuals are on the lookout for the effective means of relieving stress without even realizing that they naturally have one of the best stress relievers and that is breathing. Breathing exercises do not just relax your mind and body but these are also proven to boost your immune system. Experts even suggest that individuals should take a deep breath whenever negative thoughts and feelings strike in.

Breathing

It was found out that breathing exercises have a profound effect on health. Individuals who take time to perform these types of exercises especially during stressful times feel a lot better than those who do not do breathing exercises.

Studies were conducted and it was found out that breathing exercises alter the blood's PH and change blood pressure. Most importantly these exercises can be utilized as methods of training the reaction of the body towards stressful situations and dampen and reduce the production of risky stress hormones. Rapid breathing is said to be controlled by the human sympathetic Nervous System. This is part of flight or fight response, the part which is activated by stress. To relieve stress, deep and slow breathing is necessary.

Breathing exercises are crucial for ultimate recovery from stress and depression. Making deep breaths stimulate the PNS or Parasympathetic Nervous System which is responsible for various activities occurring when the body is at complete rest. The following are the most suggested breathing exercises that individuals can try to relieve anxiety, depression and stress and the surprising benefits that individuals can get should they decide to perform these exercises:

Coherent Breathing

This is a type of breathing exercise at a rate of 5 breaths every minute. This is said to be the middle of the rate range of resonant breathing. This is done by making five inhales and five exhales. This breathing rate aids in maximizing Heart Rate Variability or HRV, which is defined as the rate of performance of PNS. A change in pattern and rate of breathing can alter HRV causing shifts in the nervous system. The higher the Heart Rate Variability or HRV is better because this entails a healthier cardiovascular system and stronger response system for stress.

Resistance Breathing

Resistance breathing exercise is breathing by creating resistance to the ideal flow of air. Resistance can be made by pursuing your lips, placing your tongue's tip against the inner and upper teeth, and hissing to your clenched teeth. You also must tighten your throat muscles, close the glottis partly and narrow spaces between your vocal cords with the aid of an external object like straw.

Breath Moving

This is when breathing moves complementary to your imagination. An expert compared this breathing exercise to a deep internal massage. It is as if allowing your breath to take a short journey to your entire body. As an example, when you are breathing, imagine that you can move your breath to your head, spine, sit bones and other parts of the body. This can somehow give you relaxation and relieve the stress you are feeling.

Individuals got the power to change the pattern and rate of their breathing deliberately. Scientific studies proved that controlling breaths helps in managing stress and all other stress-related conditions. Breath control and breathing exercises are not just used as a stress reliever. These are also utilized in other practices like tai chi, yoga, and meditation.

Many individuals these days are embracing breathing exercises to reduce stress and promote relaxation. Aside from these, breathing exercises also play an essential role in getting rid of chest tightness, fatigue, light-headedness, faintness, panic feelings, heart palpitations and more. The following are the benefits you can get when you perform breathing exercises to reduce and eliminate stress:

- Breathing exercises to relieve stress work quickly.
- Individuals who feel exhausted and stressed can perform these exercises anytime, anywhere.
- No professional skills and intense practice are required to master these exercises.
- One of the most amazing benefits of breathing exercises is that that they are free.
- Individuals who are stressed can perform these exercises even amid stressful scenarios to stay relaxed and calm.

- Breathing exercises can efficiently reverse an individual's stress response avoiding the unwanted effects and impacts of chronic stress.

Use Reminders

When individuals are stressed and confused, the tendency is for them to lose focus on things and events that they are attending to. There are many ways on how to rectify this issue and using reminders is one of them. There are instances that individuals tend to look for great solutions without knowing that by just simply using reminders, they are getting closer to a happy and stress-free way of living. The following are simple yet powerful reminders that individuals should think about especially if life is throwing little doses of difficulty and stress:

Reminders

Happiness is not constant. You must remind yourself that you will certainly have to overcome bad and stressful days because not every day is a happy day. You are not guaranteed lifetime happiness because this is believed to be the only series of great moments that adds sweetness and beauty to life. However, it is your choice if you want to stay happy or stressed. You still must keep in mind that there are still inevitable instances in life that can happen beyond your control, and these can interfere with your happiness.

Failures are considered temporary scenarios. Failure to achieve or accomplish something is not a reason to be stressed out and devastated. You must be reminded that failures are only temporary, and these are meant to teach you necessary lessons in life. Remember that the best lessons in life are learned from the worst mistakes and darkest hours of life. It is true that individuals fail at times but the quicker you accept your failure, the better person you become. Individuals are never a hundred per cent sure about the things waiting in line and this makes committing failures and mistakes naturally occurring things.

Though you cannot notice it now, you are making progress. You may not be in the position or place that you wanted to be yet, but if you practise patience, determination, and personal effort, you may likely reach there. Never allow stress and negative emotions to stop you from doing what you have always wanted. You got lots of reasons to dream and believe that you can fulfil all those dreams.

Always be reminded that trusting yourself can make you feel more confident not because you have always made the right decisions and choices but because you have successfully survived all setbacks and challenges. It would not harm to cry in the event of failure but make sure that after you have released your stress and let go of your negative emotions, you will be more optimistic and determined.

The level of stress is not a real and exact measure-Being afraid does not always mean that you are in danger and being alone does not also mean that nobody cares and loves you. Always look beyond all your doubts and search for the truth. The best way to overcome stress is to get rid of negative thoughts and actions and develop positive ones for these are more powerful. Go for a stress-free life and always remember that you must let go of how you unpleasantly feel, look forward to what you truly deserve and keep moving forward. Never let stress and fears rule and define you.

Your life now is not what has been in the past. No matter how stressful and chaotic your life has been in the past, the future remains fresh, clean, and open and wide slate. You are not your previous habits, past failures and not the old person that others have treated before. You are what you are now, and you are special.

Failure to get what you want can be a blessing - Some individuals feel stressed and frustrated if they fail to get what they want. This should not be the case because this may sometimes be an amazing stroke of better opportunities. This scenario encourages individuals to re-evaluate things and go with the best choices.

CHAPTER SIX

Make Sure to Network

When you are stressed, it would be best to reach out to people because this is an excellent means of getting support from a network of friends, families, and colleagues. Make sure to network whenever you are in stressful situations because this helps ease your troubles and allow you to view things differently. Experts revealed that connecting with people give you the support you need. The activities you do with families, friends and loved ones can help you relax. Even a simple laugh with them can be a fantastic stress reliever.

Network

Making a network is synonymous with making connections and this is essential in terms of relieving stress and establishing better relationships. Getting an ideal social support system from family, peers and friends provides the feeling of comfort and security, knowing that you are not alone in your stressful struggle. The following are the benefits you will get when you network and create connections:

The feeling of Ideal Security

Social networks provide individuals with access to guidance, pieces of advice and assistance that they need. It is quite a relief to know that you have someone to count on in times of need.

Increased Self-Confidence

Having many people around you is an implication that you are such a nice person to spend time with. Having enough support from individuals who matters a lot to you make you feel more confident about overcoming stress and all other problems.

Sense of Belonging

Reaching out and spending time with others ease stress and loneliness. Whether it is with your siblings, buddies, and friends, knowing that you are not alone can help you cope with stress. To eliminate stress, make sure to network and create ideal connections to reap more benefits such as feeling less isolated, judged, and lonely, gaining a sense of control and empowerment, improving coping skills and adjustment, talking honestly and openly about feelings, and lastly reducing anxiety and stress.

Networking is getting to know other people more. It might be unknown to you, but you are already doing networking every single day. You are networking when you start a conversation with others or introduce yourself to groups, meet a friend, catch up with former workmates and more. Your attention is being diverted to positive things leaving no room for stress.

Get the "I Will Be Calm" Mentality

Stress can affect individuals in varying ways, but they are fortunate enough because there are many things, they can do about this. Embracing the "I Will be Calm" mentality is one effective way of coping with stress. There are several ways to calm down instantly when you are overwhelmed and blindsided by stress suddenly. The following are easy and quick ways to regain calmness during stressful situations.

Taking a Walk

Exercising is an excellent stress reliever because this helps in blowing off steam and releasing endorphins. Taking a walk when you are stressed out can provide you with the benefit of both long- and short-term exercises. This takes you out of the stressful situation and provides you with a new perspective and frame of mind. Walking with a close relative and friend is also a helpful way to get support. However, walking alone is also good because this gives individuals time to reframe and re-evaluate things.

Taking a Deep Breath

As part of embracing calmness mentality, taking a deep breath is essential. Doing breathing exercises when you are trapped within stressful situations can help you feel better. Getting more amount of oxygen in the body and releasing tension are just a few of the many benefits you can get when you do breathing exercises.

Taking Mental Break

If you are given the chance to escape from a busy and stressful world, grab it. This can give you genuine moments of visualization and peace of mind. Taking a mental break is also an ideal means of relaxing mentally and physically. Get access to a happy place and be ready to enjoy a calm of stress-free life.

Finding Pleasure

When stress bothers you and makes you feel worst, engage in activities that will make you feel good. Find pleasure in simple things to help you get rid of stress. You can plan an art project, find a new hobby, read books and magazines, play your favourite sport, listen to beautiful music and many more.

Reframing Situations

Sometimes, individuals complicate things because they view stressful situations as things that are difficult to deal with. Reframing situations is therefore a helpful way of regaining calmness. Look at your situations differently to gain new perspectives and with that, you are getting closer to a stress-free life. As much as possible, practice the act of calmness and patience and avoid pessimistic things that sabotage you from fulfilling your goals.

Relaxing Muscle

Relaxing your muscle can also be an effective and helpful technique that helps in releasing tension. By using the right approach and means of relaxing your muscle, you can completely release all the stress and tension you are feeling. Once you have already calmed down, you will notice that you will be in a better position to deal with any stressful situations you will encounter. It is also a brilliant idea to implement and adopt regular stress slayer and healthy habits for the overall reduction of stress so that you will be less bothered. Embracing the "I Will be Calm" mentality is a crucial addition to your resolution list.

www.ingramcontent.com/pod-product-compliance
Lightning Source LLC
Chambersburg PA
CBHW031922270726
48655CB00007BA/3203